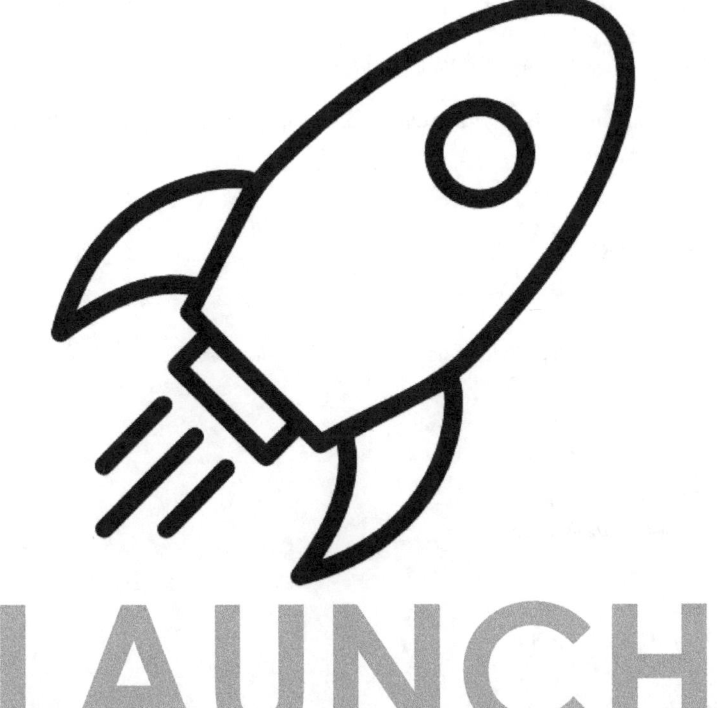

# LAUNCH

## ANDREW EDWIN JENKINS

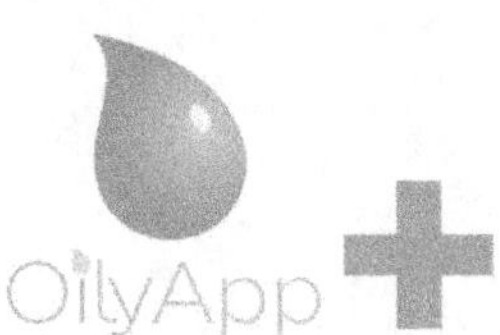

YOUR FLIGHT PLAN
FROM STARTER KIT
TO SUCCESS
IN JUST 10 WEEKS

**For more info about this title, video content, and more, go to www.OilyApp.com/launch (URL is case-sensitive).**


**Connect online!**

**Podcast-**
OilyApp, available on Apple Podcasts, Google, Stitcher, or your favorite provider.

**Social-**
www.Facebook.com/OilyApp
www.Facebook.com/OilyApp
www.Instagram.com/OilyApp

**YouTube-**
www.YouTube.com/OilyApp

**Website-**
OilyApp.com

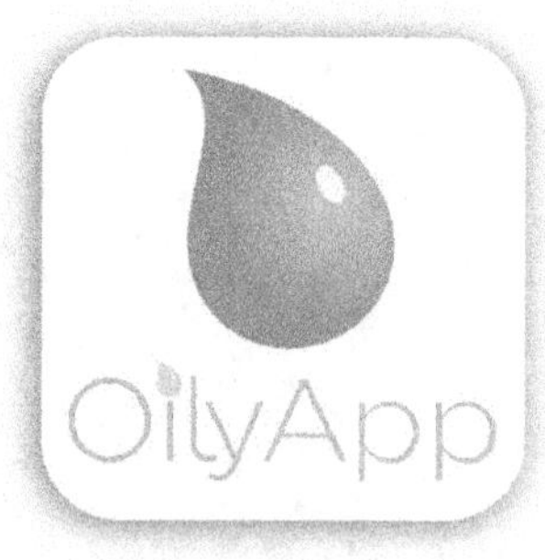

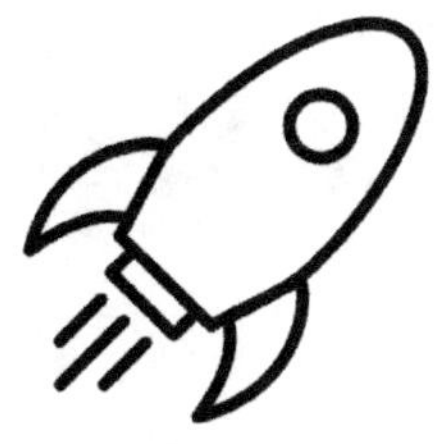

# CONTENTS



## YOUR FIRST TEN WEEKS

# APPENDIX

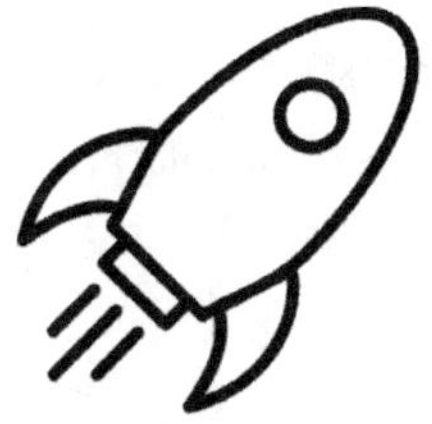

# FROM STARTER KIT
# TO SUCCESS

We created OilyApp (go to OilyApp.com to learn more) with the goal of educating you about Young Living's vast array of incredible products. The app is uniquely the *only* third party app that's an approved partner of Young Living Essential Oils, passing a strict compliance review each time we update.

OilyApp works well with Young Living's stated mission of taking oils into every home in the world. Once people have the oils, *they need to know how to use them.*

Whereas shipping a desk reference to everyone is cumbersome and difficult (besides, who wants to always lug it around!?), most people have a smart phone. An app is the perfect solution.

Furthermore, our app does other things books can't do. When Young Living releases a new product, we don't do a reprint– we simply push a notification to people who paid the one-time fee to purchase the app. And, you can manage your personal inventory, create wish lists, watch videos, and access other training tools, as well- all impossibilities with a book.

(Once again, the total irony of reading all of that in a book isn't lost on me.)

Furthermore, the app was created by actual members (Ernie and his wife, Myra, are Royal Crown Diamonds, the highest rank in the company). That is, our founder created the app in the field for use in the field.

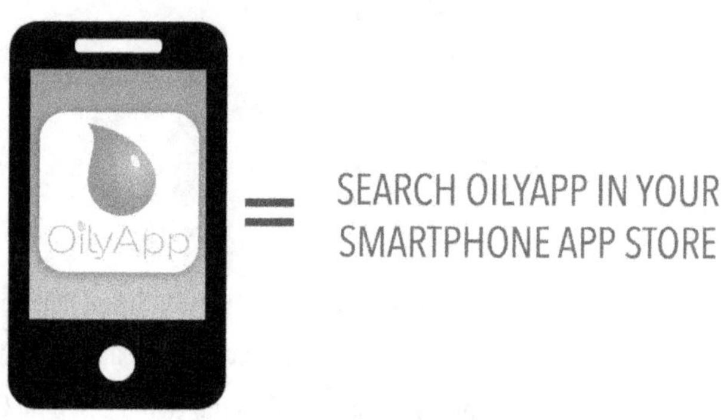


## *WHERE OUR BOOKS CAME FROM—*

After a few years of providing users with OilyApp, it became apparent that another addition was needed for product users and business builders who wanted to go to the "next level." Enter OilyApp+, a web-based experience designed to provide users with more relevant information— things like scripts they could use to learn and/or educate their teams, graphics that were relevant and educational, and videos that provide deep-dive training.

(You can take a deep-dive about OilyApp+ at OilyApp.com/plus.)

We created OilyApp+ in *less than two weeks* from its conception.

From the beginning, we knew we wanted the OA+ to include video courses and online scripts– tools you could use to review and then teach your "people" what you were learning.

After a few weeks, the thought hit us: *What if we made the scripts into small books, too– small pocket-sized books people could easily review and use to study, to lead others, and even to teach classes?*

We wrote…

… and then wrote some more.

And, we continued writing and creating…

Hence the title you have in your hand, #14 in our series.

---

## THE CHANGE-UP

But this book is a bit different than the others we've released. Whereas most of our previous books try to teach you about the products, this book provides you with a map to navigate your way *through* those products.

Let's face it. The world of essential oils and natural health can be, well, overwhelming. There's so much information out there– in the form of printed pages, websites, and even smartphone apps.

*Where do you begin?*

*And then where do you go from there?*

*And where are we even going?*

You might feel– like us– that you could use a proven strategy to help you get "lift off" in this new essential oil habit. Whether you're looking to boost your health or even take a look at the biz opportunity, we've got you covered.

*Launch* is your map to move from here to there, using simple steps that have worked for others and will– guaranteed– work for you, too.

(By the way, this course is also *perfect* to share with your friends who are new to this thing, too!)

---

## OUR GOAL

You might find it helpful to read this entire book cover to cover immediately, but *Launch* is designed to serve as a companion, your guide, for the next 10 weeks.

Here's what the book will do:

**EQUIP** YOU WITH AN ON-RAMP FOR YOUR FIRST 10 WEEKS

**EXPLORE** THE WORLD OF ESSENTIAL OILS

**EXPOSE** YOU TO OIL-INFUSED PRODUCTS RELATED TO THINGS YOU DO

**EMPOWER** YOU TO KNOW WHERE TO GO WHEN YOU NEED SOMETHING

**EDUCATE** YOU ENOUGH TO KNOW HOW TO EDUCATE YOURSELF

**ENCOURAGE** YOU ON AS YOU BEGIN THIS JOURNEY

As such, I encourage you to locate the online videos which accompany this book if you haven't already done so. They're available at OilyApp.com/launch, as is the bundle of books we reference throughout this material.

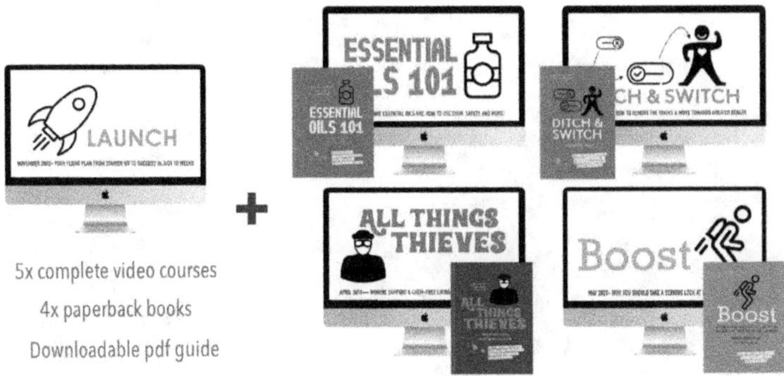

5x complete video courses
4x paperback books
Downloadable pdf guide

Whereas the books in the bundle do have a nominal cost, the podcast episodes based on them are free. URLS are provided for each throughout this book whenever we refer to them.

Whether this is the 14th book of ours you've read or the 1st, welcome.

*All the best,*

Andy

November 2020

# YOUR FIRST TEN WEEKS

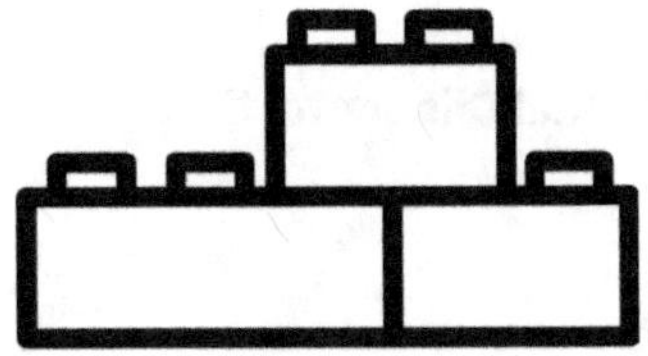

# 1. BASICS FIRST

Depending on which kit you purchased (generally, people grab the Essential Oils Premium Starter Kit or the Thieves option), we'll steer you towards a few educational resources (you can read, watch, or listen!), and we'll make sure you get connected with the right people lickety-split!

(This is the most structured week of all, as there's some foundational info we want to relay to you, to empower you on this journey.)

---

*DAY 1*

We refer to "Day 1" as the day you purchase your kit. We suggest you begin with either the Essential Oils Premium Starter Kit or the Thieves Starter Kit.

(If you don't yet have a kit, refer to the person who gave you this book for ordering info. If you stumbled upon this, PM/DM @OilyApp on Instagram or Facebook.)

Depending on which kit you purchased, **_do the following today_** (even if you are awaiting your kit to arrive in the mail)…

**If you ordered the Essential Oils Starter Kit…**

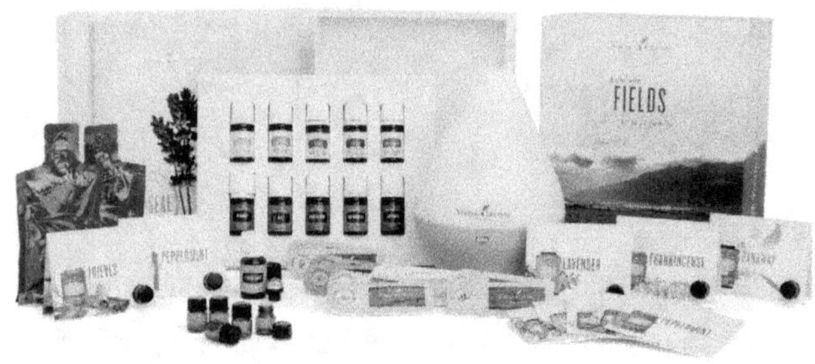

- [ ] Read *Essential Oils 101* (about 120 pages, with lots of pictures). It will take about 2 hours to read it, so plan to finish it this week.

- [ ] Watch the video class for Essential Oils 101 *or* listen to the podcast episodes where it's taught (episodes 67, 68, 69)

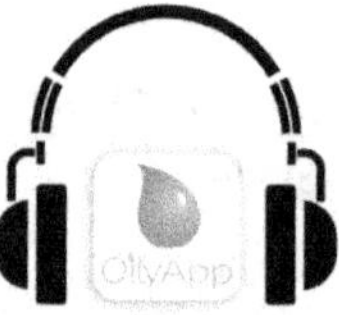

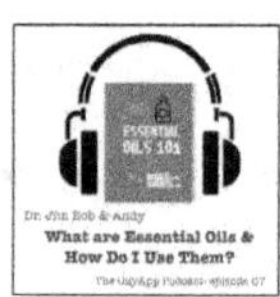


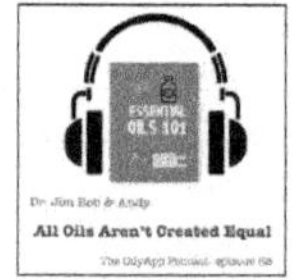


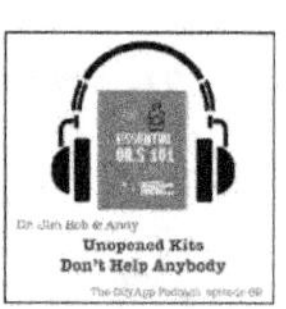


PODCAST EPISODES 67, 68, 69

☐ Find the free 21 Day Challenge at www.OilyApp.com/101. Again, sign up for this challenge day you order your kit (even if you need to wait a few days to arrive in the mail).

Note: the 21 Day Challenge is also in chapter 5 of the 101 book if you prefer a printed version.

**IF YOU ORDERED THE PREMIUM STARTER KIT (ESSENTIAL OILS)**

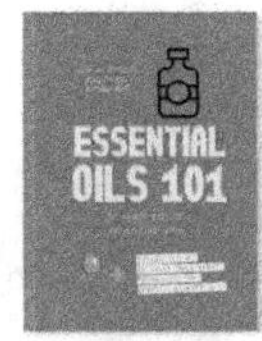
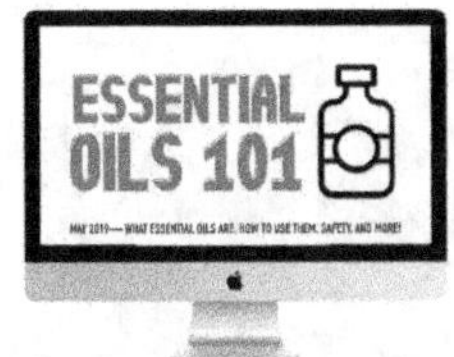
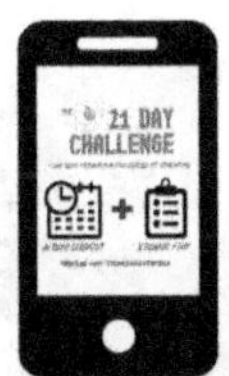

## READ

**ESSENTIAL OILS 101**

## LOOK/LISTEN

**PODCAST + VIDEO COURSE**

## DO

**21 DAY CHALLENGE**

## If you ordered the Thieves Kit...

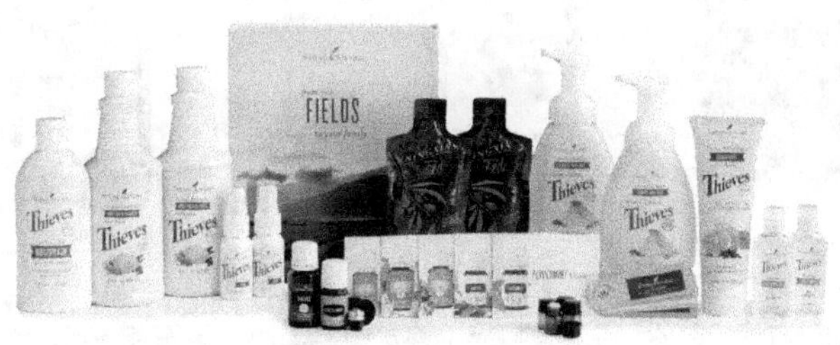

☐ Read *All Things Thieves* (about 120 pages, great graphics, takes about 2 hours of total time to work through).

☐ Watch the *All Things Thieves* class *or* listen to the podcast episodes where it's taught (episodes 70, 71, 72, 73).

☐ Review the "67 Legit Uses for Thieves" from chapter 7 of the *All Things Thieves* book.

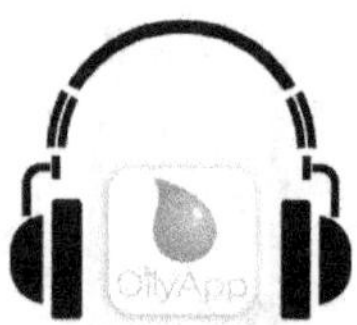
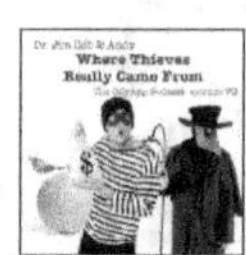
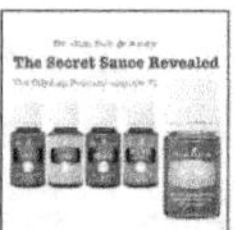
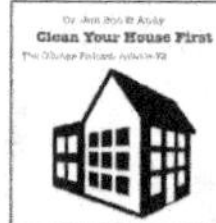
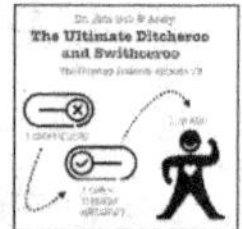

**PODCAST EPISODES 70, 71, 72, 73**

Notice, *the tasks are very similar for each kit.* You'll read a short book + watch a few videos or listen to a few talks.

**IF YOU ORDERED THE THIEVES STARTER KIT**

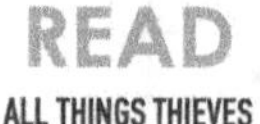

| READ | LOOK/LISTEN | DO |
|---|---|---|
| ALL THINGS THIEVES | PODCAST + VIDEO COURSE | 67 USES FOR THIEVES |

---

## DAY 2

Open whichever kit you have– if you've not already done so. Here's the task for today:

☐ Verify you have each of the items that are included with your kit purchase.

This sounds like a "no-brainer," but you'd be surprised how many people never open the kit and explore what's there. Or how many people assume they're missing something because they can't locate the "secret compartment" in the oils box. You paid good, hard-earned cash for what Young Living sent your way– go ahead and see what you've got.

Remember, that 21 Day Challenge will take you through the oils kit. *Continue* this 3-week process if you've ordered this kit.

If you purchased Thieves, make note of the uses in the final chapter of the book– and set a time this week to do "one room at a time," *using* the Thieves products in place of what you've been using (i.e., do the laundry with Thieves, clean the kitchen with Thieves, replace your mouthwash and toothpaste with the Thieves alternatives).

---

## DAY 3

Login to your virtual office (VO) at YoungLiving.com. Hopefully, you wrote your username + password somewhere for safe-keeping when you made your purchase!

The VO is where you place future orders, locate incredible educational resources, and even launch a business if you decide to do so in the future.

Today, I want you to do a few things:

- ☐ Find the link with your member number embedded in it. It will be long and cumbersome. I've placed mine in the footnote below, so you can see what one looks like.[1]

- ☐ Take a picture of you with your open box– don't think too hard about staging it, just shoot it with your phone.

- ☐ Post that image to social media.

For your caption, tell everyone something like, "Hey, just started this journey making some healthier choices for me + my family. No worries, I'm not going to turn my social media feed into an infomercial for Young Living. But, if you have questions or want to join me on this journey, send me a PM or hit the link in the comments."

Then, be sure to just paste that long link *in the comments* of your post, so that if someone makes a purchase it goes to your credit– and no worries if no one does. You're just breaking the ice here, not trying to launch a million dollar biz.

Note: you're going to begin posting on social media at least once a day (6 days a week). But, you're only going to mention your products about once out of those 6 days.[2]

--------

[1] https://www.youngliving.com/vo/#/signup/new-start?
sponsorid=20272274&enrollerid=20272274&isocountrycode=US&culture=en-US&type=member

[2] If you're itching to learn more about social media, go ahead and review chapter 9.

## DAY 4

Make sure you drop in all of the Facebook groups (or chat threads) your upline has.

Here's space to write the name of those groups if you need to make a few phone calls or send a few messages to find out where they are.

_______________________________________________

_______________________________________________

_______________________________________________

_______________________________________________

Some leaders have text threads and message bots that can send you info, too. While you're checking into online groups, ask about these, too.

_______________________________________________

_______________________________________________

Be sure to connect with us online at Facebook.com/OilyApp.

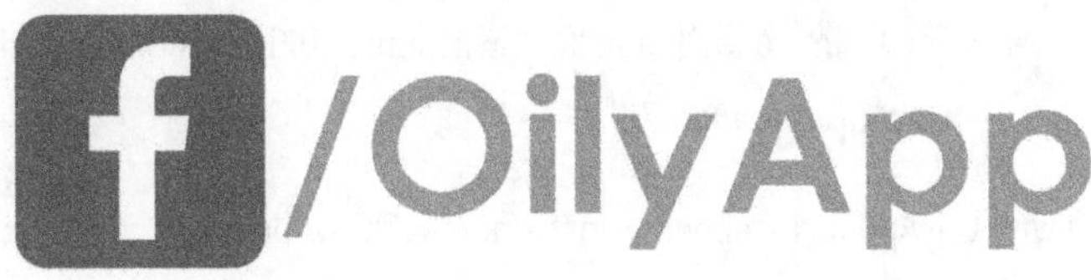

---

## IMPORTANT LINKS THIS WEEK

Essential Oils 101 course = OilyApp.com/101

Podcasts related to Essential Oils 101

- What are essential oils & how do I use them? (Essential Oils 101 #1), OilyApp.com/blog/67

- Quality issues, oil popularity, and mass confusion (Essential Oils 101 #2), OilyApp.com/blog/68

- Overcome "sealed kit syndrome" (Essential Oils 101 #3), OilyApp.com/blog/69

- The 21 Day challenge (email): OilyApp.com/ThinkInsideTheBox

Our "All Things Thieves" course = OilyApp.com/AllThingsThieves

Podcasts about Thieves:

- Where Thieves really came from (All Things Thieves #1), OilyApp.com/blog/70

- The secret sauce revealed (All Things Thieves #2), OilyApp.com/blog/71

- Clean your house first (All Things Thieves #3), OilyApp.com/blog/72

- The Ultimate Ditcheroo and Switcheroo (All Things Thieves #4), OilyApp.com/blog/73

Connect with OilyApp on Facebook + Instagram = @OilyApp

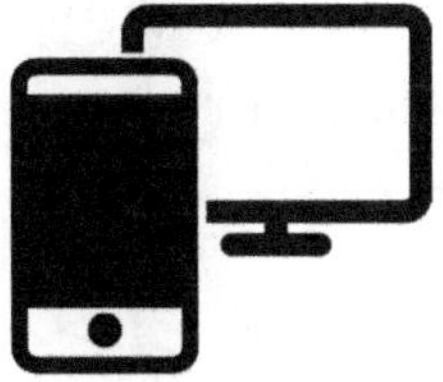

# 2. YOUR VIRTUAL OFFICE

This week you'll discover the radical program Young Living has which gives you free products every month while *also* letting you stack points you can use towards *more* free items (of your choice) in the future. Yes, we're talking Essential Rewards, YL's optional frequent buyer program.

## ESSENTIAL REWARDS

### FREQUENT BUYER PROGRAM
### POINTS BACK
### IN ADDITION TO 24% OFF
### CANCEL ANYTIME
### PRODUCTS YOU CHOOSE

This week we'll provide you with some free resources that show you how this program is different than all others, as well as show you how to leverage it to maximize your budget *and* improve your family's health.

Here's the first task of the week:

- [ ] Login to your virtual office (VO) and set up your Essential Rewards (ER) order for the *next* calendar month. (You won't be charged for the order until it ships, and you can cancel it anytime– but go ahead and get it set.)

I've written about ER and why it's important (big discounts, free products, etc.) in our *Ditch & Switch* book, which we'll study more in-depth *next* week.

While you're in the VO, order the "other kit" than what you already have. If you have an oils kit, order Thieves. If you have Thieves, order the oils.

Set your order date for next month (ER allows you to choose your processing date), so it will arrive 25-30 days from now.

The next task is to review two podcasts episodes which reference ER:

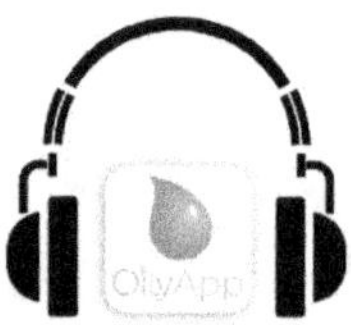

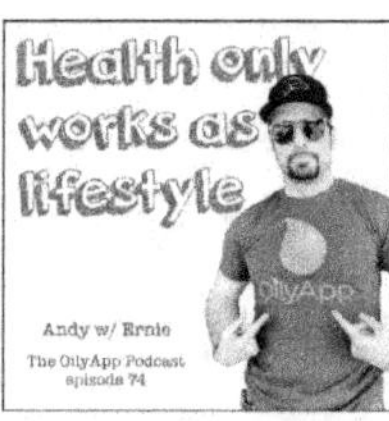


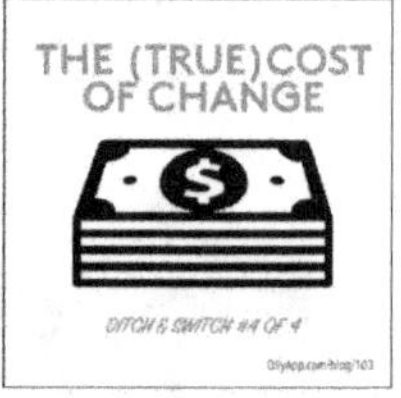


**#74**
OilyApp.com/blog/74

**#103**
OilyApp.com/blog/103

- [ ] Listen to episode 74 of the OilyApp podcast, "Health only works as a lifestyle." In this episode, Ernie chat about ER as a tool for managing your health. You can find this talk on Apple Podcasts or OilyApp.com/blog/74.

☐ Listen to episode 103, The (True) Cost of Change (Ditch & Switch #4). Find it at OilyApp.com/blog/103.

Remember to continue the 21 Day Challenge if you're studying the oils kit, or work through the "67 Legit Uses for Thieves" if you're currently learning that kit.

---

## IMPORTANT LINKS THIS WEEK

Podcast episodes related to Essential Rewards + healthy living

- Health only works as a lifestyle, OilyApp.com/blog/74

- The (True) Cost of Change (Ditch & Switch #4)- OilyApp.com/blog/103

21 Day Challenge for the oils kit = OilyApp.com/ThinkInsideTheBox

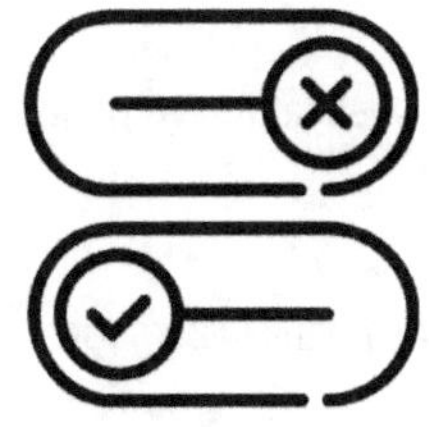

# 3. HOW TO DITCH & SWITCH

If you're around the wonderful world of Young Living for any time at all, you'll hear the phrase "Ditch and Switch."

It means this: REMOVE the toxins from your home (that is, ditch them) and IMPROVE the quality of your health by switching to healthier alternatives.

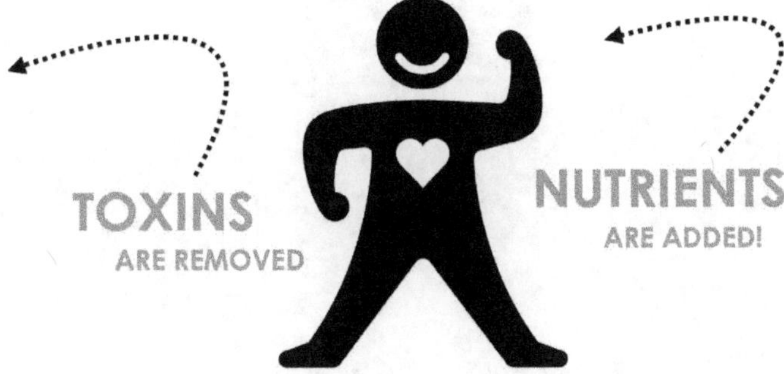

We'll show you how to use "budget dollars" for this, too– and may even SAVE you money in the process.

There are two things to do this week (along with the 21 Day Challenge, etc., which you should finish this week).

☐ Read the *Ditch & Switch* book (120 pages, lots of pictures).

Here's the premise of the book: Health really is simple– but we're more likely come be poisoned or toxified in our homes than outside of them. And, manufacturers and governments regulations mitigate *against* health. Thankfully, you can do your own research, make wise decisions, and switch unhealthy products for health alternatives. This book shows you how to understand what you're up against, uncover the benefits of change, and then make the transition as painlessly– and economically– as possible.

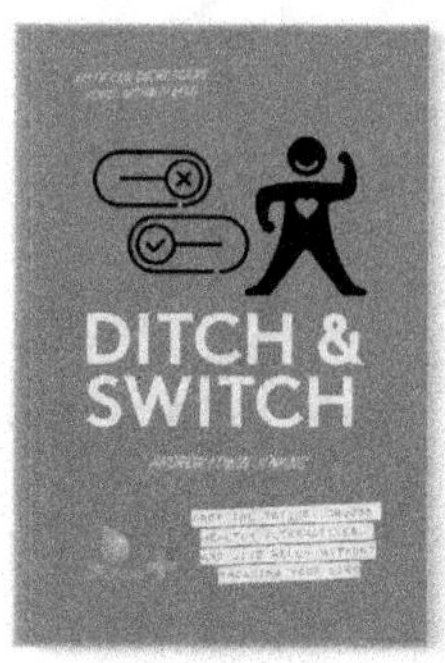


☐ Watch the Ditch & Switch course at OilyApp.com/switch or listen to the four episodes (about 20-minutes each) of the podcast series:

- Greenwashed (Ditch & Switch #1)- www.OilyApp.com/blog/100

- The Slick Seven– 1, 2, 3 (Ditch & Switch #2)- www.OilyApp.com/blog/101

- The Slick Seven– 4, 5, 6, 7 (Ditch & Switch #3)- www.OilyApp.com/blog/102

- The (True) Cost of Change (Ditch & Switch #4)- www.OilyApp.com/blog/103

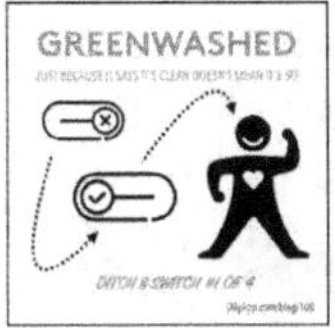

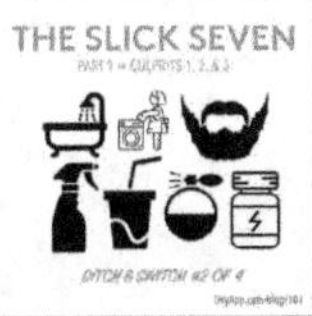

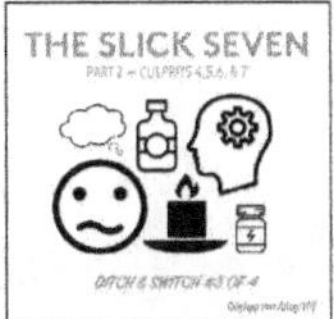

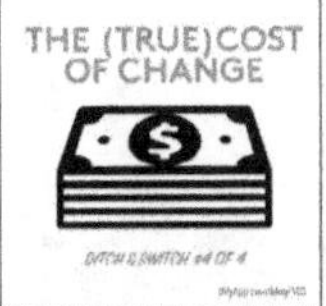


PODCAST EPISODES 100, 101, 102, 103

☐ Finally, schedule a Zoom call with your upline. Even if the call needs to happen next week, get it on the calendar now.

The purpose of this call is to communicate with someone who is a few steps ahead of you on the health + wellness journey. Ideally, your upline will have connected with you by now. But, if they haven't, just reach out. Everyone is busy, and since your health is your responsibility (and not theirs), go ahead and take the initiative.

(We'll schedule another call during week 7).

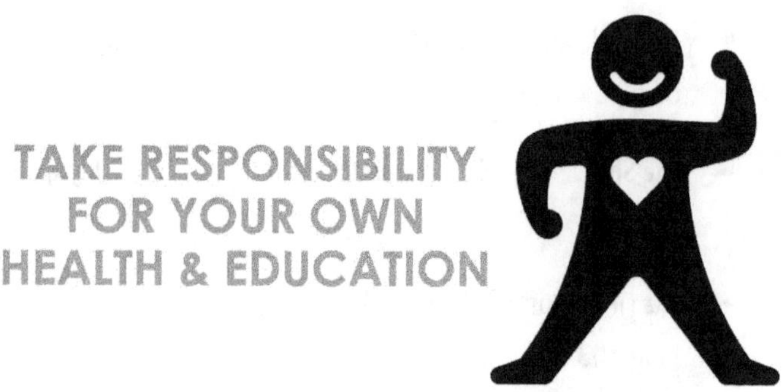


## LINKS FOR THIS WEEK

Find the Ditch & Switch course at www.OilyApp.com/switch

Listen to the four podcast episodes at:

- Greenwashed (Ditch & Switch #1)- www.OilyApp.com/blog/100

- The Slick Seven– 1, 2, 3 (Ditch & Switch #2)- www.OilyApp.com/blog/101

- The Slick Seven– 4, 5, 6, 7 (Ditch & Switch #3)- www.OilyApp.com/blog/102

- The (True) Cost of Change (Ditch & Switch #4)- www.OilyApp.com/blog/103

# 4. THE (OPTIONAL) BIZ SIDE

You probably said you weren't interested in this…

… and you may have sworn up and down, taken an oath, and even pledged in some absurd way that you would never– never, ever!– "do the business."

*Pause.*

Take a deep breathe.

And listen…

*You do, at least, owe it to yourself to take a look at what's available.*

Whether you choose to do anything more than that is completely up to you. But, by all means, do take an honest look.

Here's what you'll discover.

First, Young Living has grown steadily over the past 25+ years (we'll beyond the life-expectancy of a network-marketing company / home-based business) because of it's passion for quality products. That means you get the best stuff on the planet delivered straight to you, regardless of what you choose to do with the biz opportunity (which, again, is always optional).

Second, if you're looking for extra spending money, hoping to add to your family's bottom line, searching for a way to give back to others, or even looking for a career shift, then this *might* be your ticket to change.

This week, we're going to learn a bit about network marketing, as well as the company's compensation plan. **Even if you're not planning to "do the business side," you owe it to yourself to take a look at the potential**.

Here are the tasks for the week:

☐ Read *Boost*, and review the compensation plan resources referenced in the book. The book is a short read (again, about 2 hours, lots of pictures), and contains great info on the products and how the healthy lifestyle works in a way that actually empowers you to grow a sustainable business without selling people stuff they don't want, don't need, or won't ever use. And, we answer all the questions (and misconceptions) people have about networking marketing.

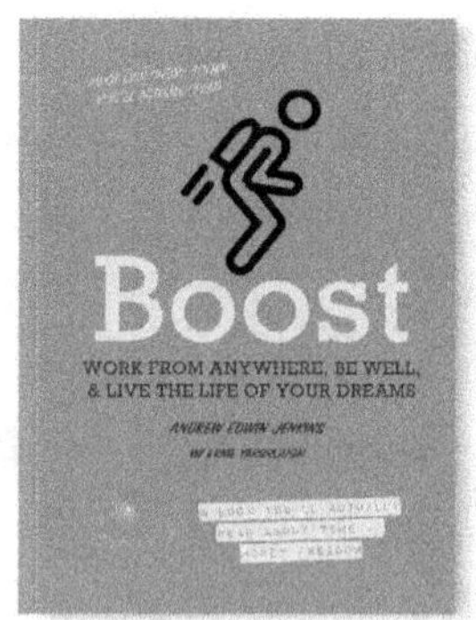

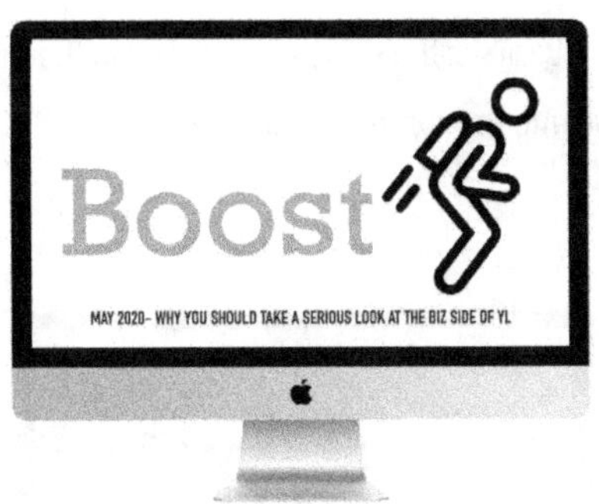



☐ Watch the Boost video course at OilyApp.com/Boost or listen to the podcast episodes related to the Boost materials:

- Stop Trading Time for Money (Boost #1), OilyApp.com/blog/87

- Four Mind Shifts You Need to Make It in This Economy (Boost #2), OilyApp.com/blog/88

- Three Secrets *They* Don't Want You to Know (Boost #3), OilyApp.com/blog/89

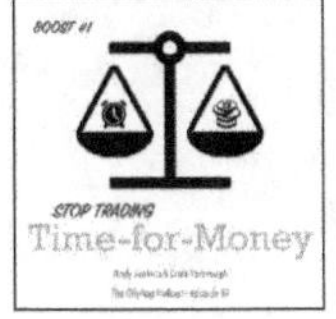



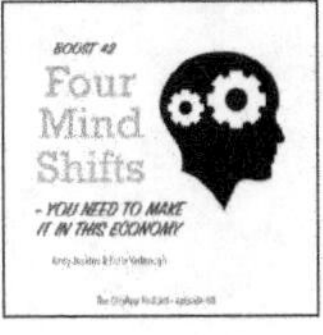

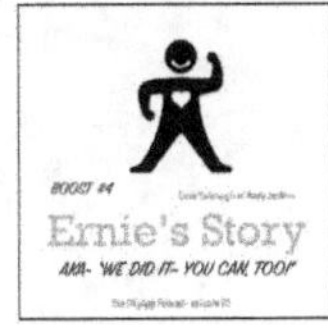

- Ernie's (Network Marketing) Story (Boost #4), OilyApp.com/blog/90

☐ Biz Building Basics is the course referenced in the materials. It takes a deeper dive into the compensation plan. Find it at OilyApp.com/biz.

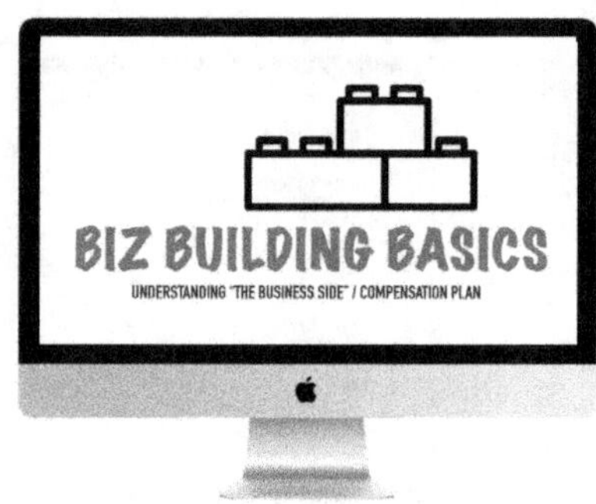


☐ Review the following links on Young Living's website:

- Income Disclosure Statement = www.YoungLiving.com/IDS

- Bridge to Gold = www.youngliving.com/en_US/opportunity/ bridge-to-gold

# LOOK AT—

## SILVER IN SIX

## BRIDGE TO GOLD

## INCOME DISCLOSURE STATEMENT AT YOUNGLIVING.COM/IDS

---

## LINKS FOR THE WEEK

The Boost video course = OilyApp.com/Boost

Podcast episodes related to Boost=

- Stop Trading Time for Money (Boost #1), OilyApp.com/blog/87

- Four Mind Shifts You Need to Make It in This Economy (Boost #2), OilyApp.com/blog/88

- Three Secrets *They* Don't Want You to Know (Boost #3), OilyApp.com/blog/89

- Ernie's (Network Marketing) Story (Boost #4), OilyApp.com/blog/90

Biz Building Basics (compensation plan course) = OilyApp.com/biz

Links on Young Living's website =

- Income Disclosure Statement = www.YoungLiving.com/IDS

- Bridge to Gold = https://www.youngliving.com/en_US/ opportunity/bridge-to-gold

# 5. YOUR NEXT KIT(S)

By now, you're one month into your essential oil journey.

You'll hear us say something like this over and over: "Health only works as a lifestyle." So, we'll provide you with a few steps to begin that journey to more + better.

This week we show you what to order next, now that you've begun using (and reaping the benefits of) your first kit.

The task for this week is simple to understand:

☐ Begin working through *your next kit* (i.e., if you began with the oils kit, move to the Thieves kit– or vice versa), as outlined on Day 1.

The 21 Day Challenge (oils kit) will take about 10 minutes per day, and the Thieves learning process will take about the same amount of time– though it['s not as structured.

Remember, you'll need the following:

- The relevant book (either *Essential Oils 101* or *All Things Thieves*)

- The video courses for each book or podcast episodes

The tasks for this week are found in chapter 1 of this book– simply do the *opposite* kit of what you did the first week.

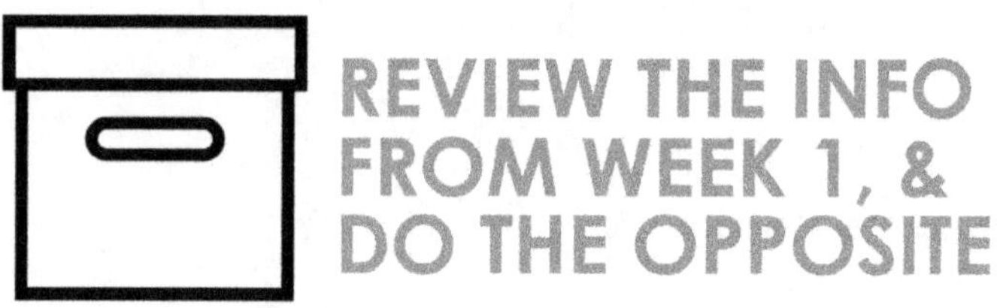

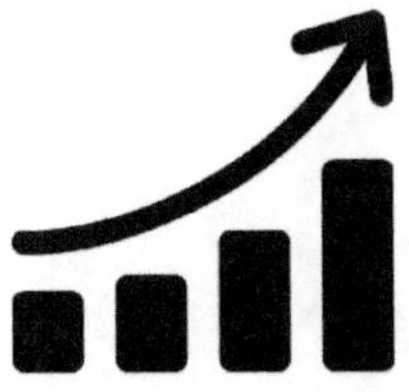

# 6. REMOVE, IMPROVE

Many great ideas fail, because there's no plan to follow through with the plan.

The *idea* of health is fabulous. And the *goal* of ditching toxins and switching to healthier alternatives is honorable. But, it's easier– and totally doable over the long-term– if you have a plan to implement it.

(On the other hand, without a plan, this goal is likely destined to fail.)

In this week of study (and in the video), we'll show you what we do, toss out a few options for you to check for yourself, and provide you with a launch pad to craft your own strategy.

- [ ] First, set up your Essential Rewards order for the following month.

  You've ordered an oils kit and a Thieves kit. This month (for your next order) try the NingXia Red kit (NingXia is a powerhouse supplement, which you drink.

- [ ] Second, learn more about NingXia by watching the video at OilyApp.com/Red.

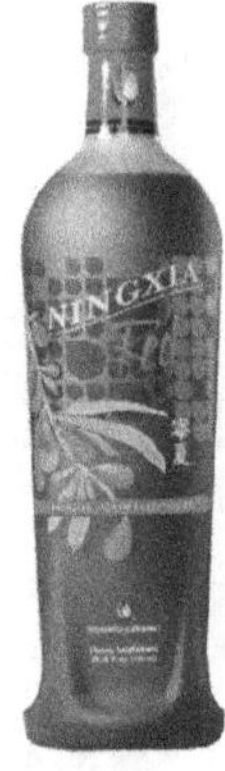


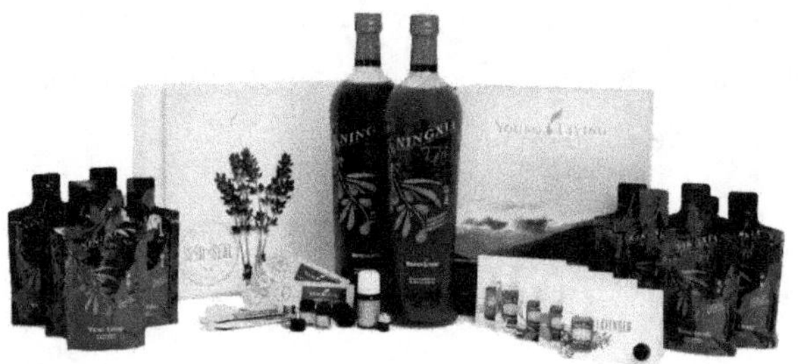

☐ Third, review chapter 12 of the Ditch & Switch book where I discuss Essential Rewards and provide you with an overview of my plan. Then, begin to create your plan. We've provided you space here if you need to make notes.

_____________________________________________

_____________________________________________

_____________________________________________

_____________________________________________

_____________________________________________

_____________________________________________

_____________________________________________

_____________________________________________

# ESSENTIAL REWARDS TIP

## MAKE A PLAN

## BUDGET YOUR PLAN

Like we discuss in the *Ditch & Switch* book, for Essential Rewards shopping we use "budget dollars" (transferring money we were planning to spend at the store to, instead, purchase healthier products at a comparable– or even better– price).

## ESSENTIAL REWARDS ISN'T JUST ONLY ACCUMULATING ESSENTIAL OILS.

## ESSENTIAL REWARDS IS ABOUT WALKING IN A LIFESTYLE OF HEALTH + WHOLENESS

In general, I order a Thieves ER kit one month, then a NingXia Red kit the following month. I alternate this every other month, adding other products I need to each month's order (i.e., oils I need to replace, personal care products, etc.). Because I'm placing orders on a 30-day cycle, I purchase these kits even if I have some product on hand. This way, I never run out.

Essential Rewards is the tool I also use to manage the supplements and foundational products I need for my overall health.

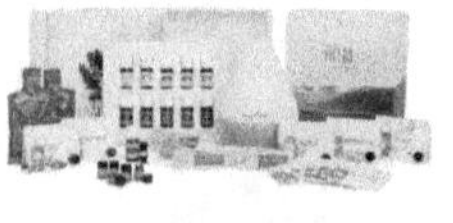

INTRO TO NATURAL HEALTH

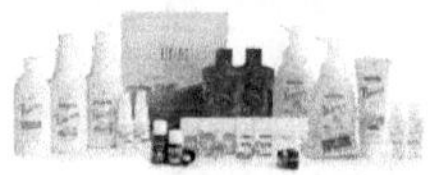

CHEMICAL/TOXIN-FREE LIVING

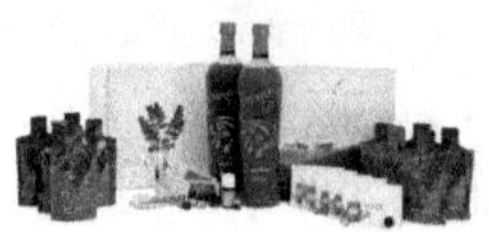

SUPPLEMENT, FULL BODY SUPPORT

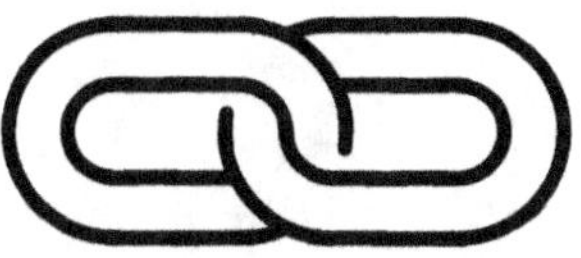

# 7. CONSTANT CONNECTION

One of the greatest assets Young Living has is the people to whom you are connected via this network of essential oil users.

- [ ] Schedule another Zoom call with your upline, to review any questions you have, discuss what you are learning, etc.

- [ ] Continue your study, catching up on any weeks where you may have fallen behind.

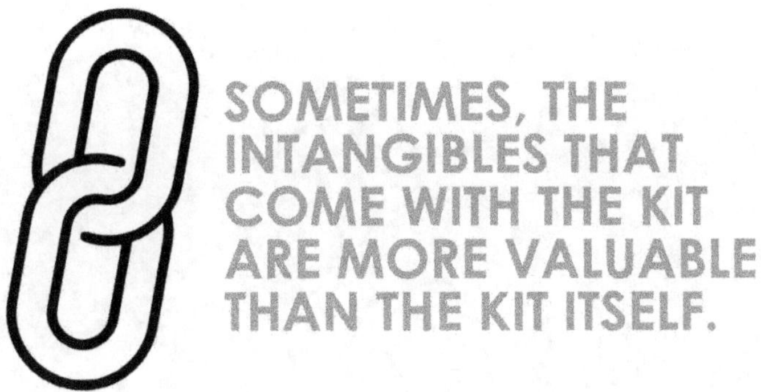

# 8. EXPLORE SOME MORE

You're probably already doing something you love, and you might be surprised to learn that essential oils can enhance that thing. This week we have a simple challenge for you…

☐ Choose one area you would like to learn more about essential oils or oil-infused products may accentuate or accelerate a current hobby or interest.

This should be ideally be something you *already* do (i.e., fitness, pets, etc.) or something you *really* want to do (i.e., lose weight).

We'll show you a few options and then provide you with a way to integrate essential oil + oil-infused products into that area of life.

Here's how to do it:

- Look ahead at week 10.

- I've listed multiple areas of interest– all of which Young Living creates products to support and enhance.

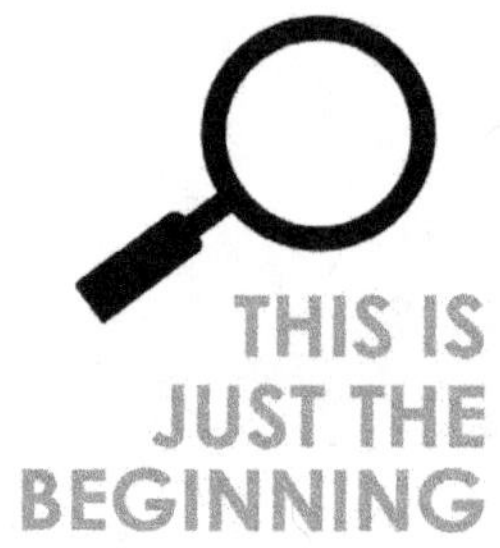

## THIS IS JUST THE BEGINNING

AGING = SUPPLEMENTS

BEAUTY = ART SKIN CARE LINE

BABIES = SEEDLINGS LINE

CBD = CBD KITS OR INDIVIDUAL PURCHASE

EMOTIONAL HEALTH = FEELINGS KIT

FITNESS = SUPPLEMENTS, ACTIVE & FIT KIT

PETS = ANIMALSCENTS LINE

PTSD = FREEDOM SLEEP & FREEDOM RELEASE

MAKEUP = SAVVY MINERALS

WEIGHT LOSS = SLIQUE KIT

SCRIPTURE = OILS OF ANCIENT SCRIPTURE

- Begin studying one of those areas now– either by reading one of the books we've referenced, watching a course, listening to a podcast series, or even studying on your own.

- This week is about exploration!

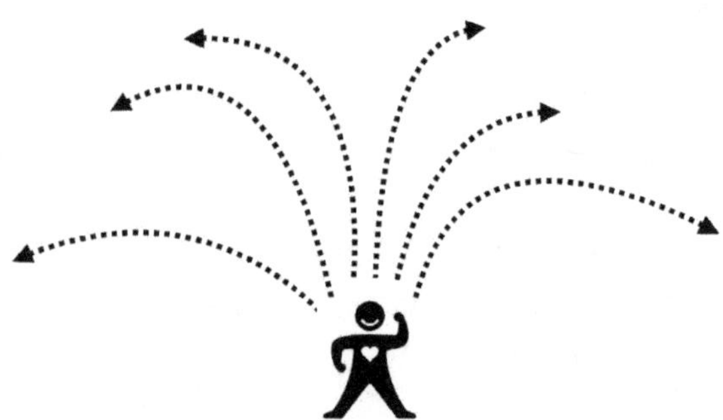

## CHOOSE YOUR OWN ADVENTURE

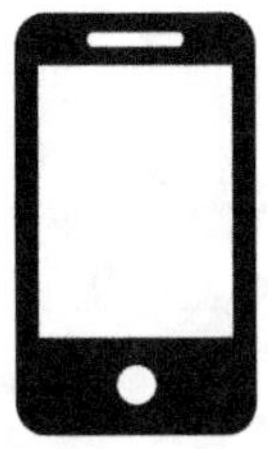

# 9. SOCIAL MEDIA 101

There are two errors you can make with social media– one is not utilizing it at all to share the products you are using. The other is over-communicating, effectively turning your social feed into one long infomercial for Young Living Essential Oils.

The mistake most people make is actually *the second*.

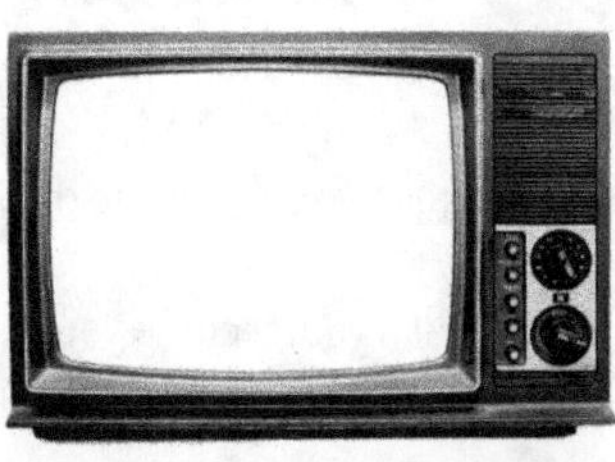



Don't turn your feeds into an infomercial. Resist the urge to copy and paste what others have written verbatim, pause before you post "one-of-a-kind blowout sale."

No, seriously.

People do it  all the time (you've probably seen it), and it can be frustrating...

We'll show you how to tip-toe the line of making *sure* you share your love of the products with others while *also* not being "that guy" that walks around with an MLM megaphone in his hand.

The launch video for week 9 is super-important if you're doing– or even checking into– the business side.

---

## CONTINUE LEARNING, AND...

This week, do the following...

- ☐ Continue your study from week 8.

- ☐ Make sure you are manage your social media feeds without turning into yet another infomercial.

Here are our suggestions on how to do that–

- Plan your feed, so you can post something to social media six days a week.

- Share something related to your YL products once a week only (if something is so great that you need to share it twice, save the second post for a future time).

- Always let people know they can PM you or leave a comment if they want more info.

- Make the posts simple– link it to something you are already doing that week (i.e., week 1 = share your box, week 2 = share something about ER and the free products you're getting, week 3 = share something you learn about the Ditch & Switch, week 4 = share something you learned from *Boost*).

- In the comments of your posts, always use your member link– the long one that has your number embedded in it. That way, if someone makes a purchase, you'll get credit.

---

## WHAT DO I POST?

I generally post twice a day– but I work online, so my rhythm is a bit different that most people's. When I spoke with a friend who was starting this journey, we created the following flow for him (and, note: he can change that as he wants. Having a plan simply prevents him from having to "come up with something" new every day.

Here's what his currently looks like:

- Sunday = off (doesn't mean he can't post, just means he doesn't feel pressured to do so)

- Monday = Share something he did from the weekend (favorite picture of the kids, something he learned at church, etc.)

- Tuesday = Something he's been reading, something he's learning (could be a quote, a picture of the page from a book, a cover of the book, etc.)

- Wednesday = Something related to Young Living (i.e., week 1 = his box… week 3 = something about Ditch & Switch, week 7 = something related to the Zoom call and walking together)

- Thursday = Music. This guy likes music, so he started sharing some of his favorite songs. (You might choose a hobby of your own.)

- Friday = Plans for the weekend.

- Saturday = Real time pic of something fun or relaxing.

**PLAN** YOUR FEED, SO YOU CAN POST 6 DAYS A WEEK

**ONCE A WEEK** POST A PIC OF A PRODUCT

**LET PEOPLE KNOW** YOU CAN HELP THEM— PLACE YOUR MEMBER NUMBER OR A MESSAGE IN THE COMMENTS, ENCORING THEM TO REACH OUT

**MAKE IT EASY FOR YOU** BY CONNECTING YOUR POSTS TO THINGS YOU'RE ALREADY DOING…

Here are a few more tips I've learned:

- When possible, share pictures. And, include people in the photo every chance you get.

- Questions are great, too (i.e., I'm reading ____________, what are you reading? Or, I'm going to the Farmer's Market this weekend, what about you?)

- Pictures don't have to be posted in real time. If you have several ideas you've gleaned from a book, for instance, space them over a few weeks.

## READY TO TRY?

In the following space, make a few notes related to your social media plan(s). Remember, you can change this at any time.

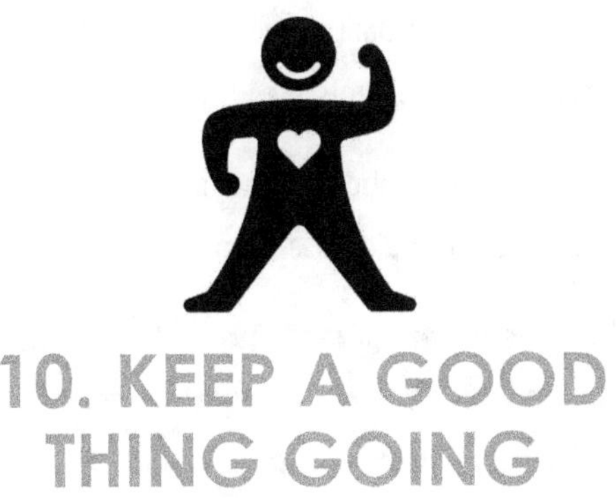

# 10. KEEP A GOOD THING GOING

*Congratulations!* You've made it all the way to chapter 10 (and week 10).

But, this is merely the end of a beginning, and it's the beginning of your next chapter…

Now, it's your time to "choose your own adventure" and integrate your essential oils + oil-infused products into your life for the long haul.

Here are the tasks for this week:

☐ Review your Essential Rewards (ER) order.

In weeks 2 and 6 week reviewed our ER order for the following month. Now, it's time to do that *again* (plan to do this every four weeks).

Each month…

1. **Alternate the kit you need** (ordering Thieves one month, NingXia the next, Thieves the next, then NingXia (I know of some people who move through entire kits in one month, so you may need to adjust your order).

2. **Determine which products you need to replace** and then add them to the order (i.e., personal care products, oils you've exhausted, supplements, etc.).

   This month add a third step, though, for this month only (can you repeat it later if you choose to do so)…

3. **Find a new area– something that's already of interest to you– in which you can integrate essential oils + natural health into your lifestyle**.

# THIS MONTH—

## ORDER THE KIT YOU NEED (THIEVES,NINGXIA RED)

## ADD PRODUCTS YOU NEED TO YOUR ORDER (I.E., PERSONAL CARE PRODUCTS, OILS YOU'VE USED, SUPPLEMENTS, ETC.)

## GO "ALL IN" ON AN AREA OF INTEREST

Here are a few options to consider:

- Aging = supplements

- Babies = Seedlings line

- CBD = CBD kits or purchase individual

- Emotional Health = Feelings Kit

- Fitness = supplements

- Pets = AnimalScents line

- PTSD = Freedom Sleep kit  & Freedom Release Kit

- Makeup = Savvy Minerals (comes as a kit or as individual products)

- Scripture = Oils of Ancient Scripture kit

- Weight loss = Slique kit

For other suggestions you can search our online video courses on our website at OilyApp.com/contents or refer to OilyApp.com/books for an updated list of print publications.

# APPENDIX

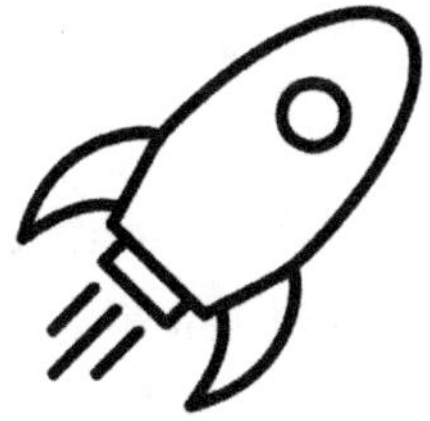

# 11. YOUR NEXT STEP

You're in one of two camps at this point in this book:

- You either already have Young Living essential oils– and are a wholesale member, *or*

- You're not one yet

If you are a wholesale member, you simply need to grab the Launch resources and begin ordering. You already have access to the products via your virtual office. strong.

If you're not a wholesale member, continue reading…

Wholesale membership doesn't tie you down to buying something every week for the rest of your life, nor does it sign you up for auto-ship or any other kind of contract… it simply means you get the prices on *the best* products… *and*, unlike Sam's or Costco where you pay a fee to become a member and have the right to shop but don't get any actual products, with Young Living you become a member when you make a purchase.

The two best options to become a wholesale member are:

- The Premium Starter Kit (aka, "essential oils" starter kit = pictured on top), or

- The Thieves Starter Kit (household products, cleaning, immune support = pictured on bottom)

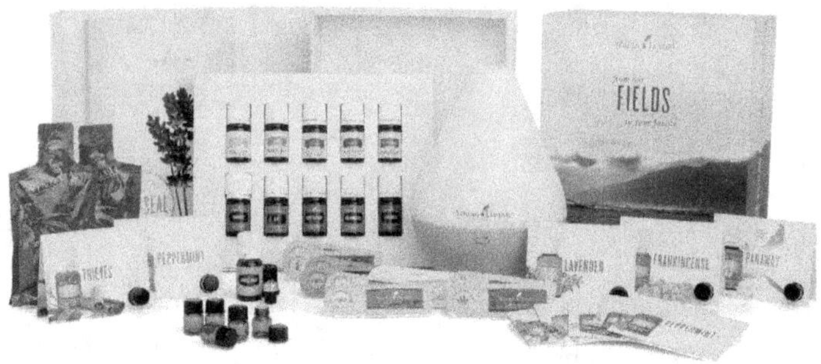

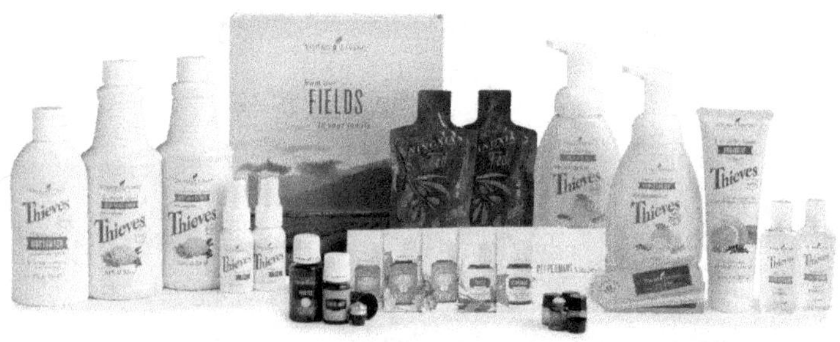

Either way you get the best products on the planet, and you can begin the Launch book study at chapter 1, week 1, day 1.

You become part of an amazing community, full of people who are learning to walk in health + wholeness. Though we come from a variety of backgrounds, we have this journey in common. And, we support one another and encourage each other through our private Facebook groups.

You'll have access to some of the best resources anywhere. With our regular calls, webinars, and online classes, you'll have great info to continue learning life-changing truths just like you're learning in this book. All of these are free to our team members.

Here's one of the best parts: wholesale members receive a 24% discount on ALL of their purchases AND they're eligible for free products every single month.

Note: if a current member offered you this book, please consult with them.

**If no one referred you, or if you took advantage of the online offer for this book, PM or DM @OilyApp on Facebook or Instagram, or call or text 205-291-1391.**

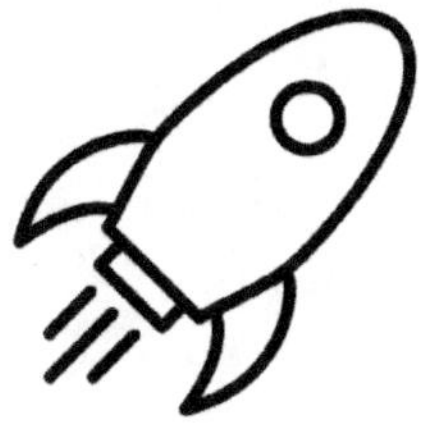

# 12. GET YOUR LEARN ON!

Each month we do the following:

- Host an online class the second Tuesday of the month. Invite friends to attend, as people who are interested in ordering will be directed to get the member link from you.

- Host an "in-person" gathering at our house on the 3rd Thursday of the month. If you're local, come to the class. We always provide food and then teach for about 25 minutes. The total time lasts about an hour– many people stay afterwards and just hang out. We stop at the 60-minute mark, so that people who need to leave can do so.

This schedule is subject to change, so verify as you make plans.

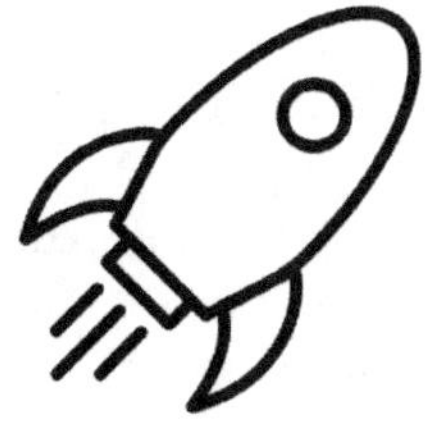

# 13. LINKS + RESOURCES

The following resources are referenced throughout this book and are placed here for easy access.

**There are four books + video courses referenced.**

Each are part of the Launch bundle, available at OilyApp.com/launch.

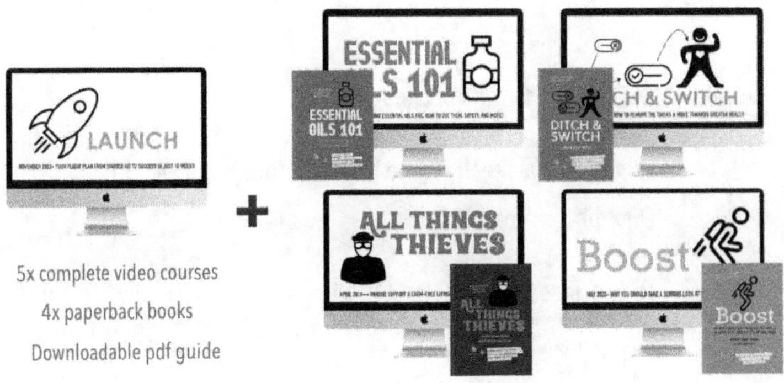


5x complete video courses
4x paperback books
Downloadable pdf guide

## Online web courses (listed in the order mentioned in this book)

- Essential Oils 101 = www.OilyApp.com/101

- All Things Thieves = OilyApp.com/AllThingsThieves

- Ditch & Switch = OilyApp.com/switch

- Boost = OilyApp.com/Boost

## Podcasts related to *Essential Oils 101*

- What are essential oils & how do I use them? (Essential Oils 101 #1), https://www.OilyApp.com/blog/67

- Quality issues, oil popularity, and mass confusion (Essential Oils 101 #2), https://www.OilyApp.com/blog/68

- Overcome "sealed kit syndrome" (Essential Oils 101 #3), https://www.OilyApp.com/blog/69

## Podcasts related to *All Things Thieves*

- Where Thieves really came from (All Things Thieves #1), OilyApp.com/blog/70

- The secret sauce revealed (All Things Thieves #2), OilyApp.com/blog/71

- Clean your house first (All Things Thieves #3), OilyApp.com/blog/72

- The Ultimate Ditcheroo and Switcheroo (All Things Thieves #4), OilyApp.com/blog/73

## Podcast episodes related to Essential Rewards + healthy living

- Health only works as a lifestyle, OilyApp.com/blog/74

- The (True) Cost of Change (Ditch & Switch #4)- OilyApp.com/blog/103

## Podcast episodes related to *Boost*

- Stop Trading Time for Money (Boost #1), OilyApp.com/blog/87

- Four Mind Shifts You Need to Make It in This Economy (Boost #2)- OilyApp.com/blog/88

- Three Secrets *They* Don't Want You to Know (Boost #3)- OilyApp.com/blog/89

- Ernie's (Network Marketing) Story (Boost #4)- OilyApp.com/blog/90

## Podcast episodes related to *Ditch & Switch*

- Greenwashed (Ditch & Switch #1)- OilyApp.com/blog/100

- The Slick Seven– 1, 2, 3 (Ditch & Switch #2)- OilyApp.com/blog/101

- The Slick Seven– 4, 5, 6, 7 (Ditch & Switch #3)- OilyApp.com/blog/102

- The (True) Cost of Change (Ditch & Switch #4)- OilyApp.com/blog/103

## Free resources / downloads

- 21 Day Challenge = OilyApp.com/ThinkInsideTheBox

- Ditch & Switch worksheet = OilyApp.com/ditchNswitch

## Other resources you need

- OilyApp = smartphone app, search in your favorite app store

- OilyApp+ = online courses, web-based, find at OilyApp.com/plus

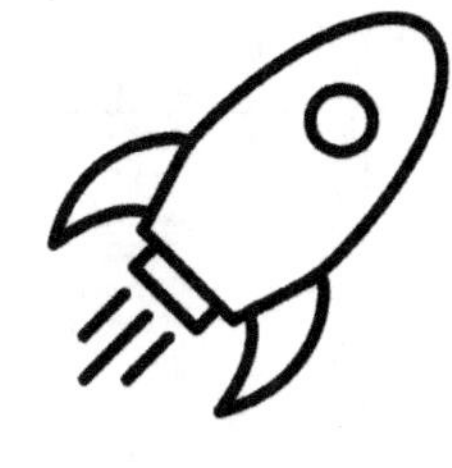

# 14. JOTS + DOODLES

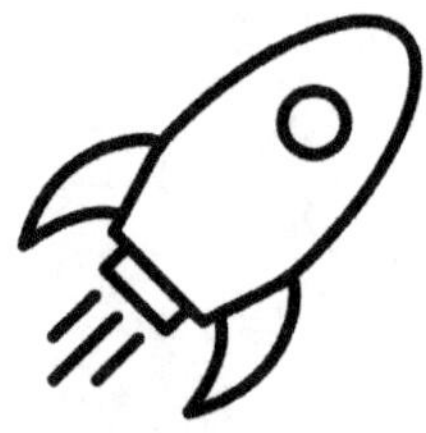

*Launch* is a bit different than the other "books you'll actually read" we've released. Whereas most of our previous books try to teach you about the products, this book provides you with a map to navigate your way *through* those products.

Let's face it: the world of essential oils and natural health can be, well, overwhelming. There's so much information out there– in the form of printed pages, websites, and even smartphone apps.

*Where do you begin?*

*And then where do you go from there?*

*And where are we even going?*

You might feel– like us– that you could use a proven strategy to help you get "lift off" in this new essential oil habit. Whether you're looking to boost your health or even take a look at the biz opportunity, we've got you covered.

*Launch* is your map to move from here to there, from starter kit to success (whatever success is to you!), using simple steps that have worked for others and will– guaranteed– work for you, too.

(By the way, this course is also PERFECT to share with your friends who are new to this thing, too!)